One Man's Victory

The story of how one man is winning the battle with Multiple Sclerosis.

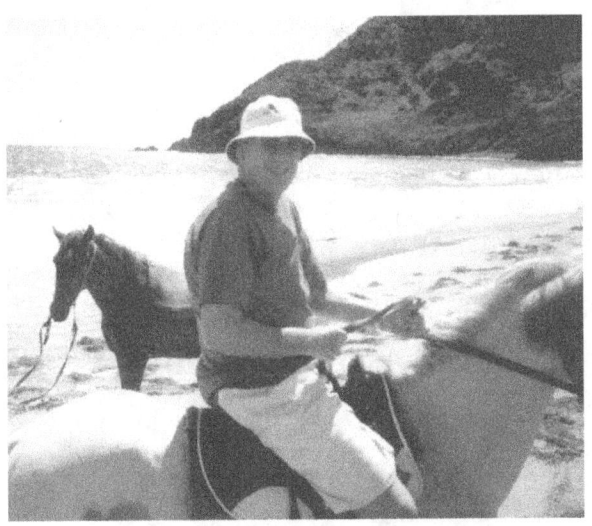

Clive Buchanan
The Lion of the Platform

Missions Publishing Inc.
P.O. Box 1537, St. George, UT 84771
Call us at 1-435-275-6649 or 1-888-344-3892
Visit Clive's website: **www.cjbuchanan.com**

The information in this book is for educational purposes only and is not recommended as a means of diagnosing or treating an illness. All matters concerning physical and mental health should be supervised by qualified health practitioners knowledgeable in treating that particular condition. Neither the publisher nor author directly or indirectly dispense medical advice, nor do they prescribe any remedies or assume any responsibility for those who choose to treat themselves.

Printed in the United States of America.

Table of Contents

Introduction
You Can Have Victory

Multiple Sclerosis (MS) is a disease or condition with few if any equals. No doctor or researcher to date has proven its cause. There are many theories. Some are very passionate about their theories but as of this writing they remain theories. If you slow, improve, or totally reverse MS you have a victory. Some victories are greater than others. I wish you total victory.

Most agree that it is in part or wholly a result of a flaw in the immune system. The body appears to attack its own nerves. There are lesions on the myelin sheath. The condition would improve if the immune system were smarter.

What is known is women are more likely to get it than men. Where you live is a factor. MS comes in several forms. Its progression and which part of the body will be affected are completely unpredictable. It affects both the physical and mental state of the victim. It is often as hard on the family as it is on the person with MS. As a group MS sufferers tend to be over-achievers. Heat and stress tend to make symptoms worse. The drugs most commonly used to treat it are marginally effective and have long lists of side effects.

Medical doctors have not researched the why and how of the program outlined in this book. But thousands have tried it and experienced improved health. The program gives you a way of thinking and nutrients that provide necessary building blocks. It is up to the body and mind to do the healing.

HOW DO YOU FEEL TODAY?

Often, we forget the little things that were bothering us before we began a nutritional program. Then, one day we suddenly realize some of those little things are no longer with us. Check the left side for those things that bother you when you start your program. At the end of 90 days, check the right side for things that have improved.

Starting Date_____ After 90 days_____

1._____	Low Energy Feel tired	1._____
2._____	Overweight	2._____
3._____	Underweight	3._____
4._____	Allergies/ Hay fever	4._____
5._____	Headaches	5._____
6._____	Splitting fingernails	6._____
7._____	Dull, thinning hair	7._____
8._____	Need stimulants to keep going	8._____
9._____	Constipation	9._____
10._____	Bleeding gums	10._____

11._____	Bruise easily	11._____
12._____	Take aspirin often	12._____
13._____	Poor digestion	13._____
14._____	Can't wake up in the morning	14._____
15._____	Can't fall asleep	15._____
16._____	High blood pressure	16._____
17._____	Depression	17._____
18._____	Aching joints	18._____
19._____	Sleep through the evening news	19._____
20._____	Skin sensitivity	20._____
21._____	Dry skin	21._____
22._____	Leg cramps	22._____
23._____	Menstrual cramps	23._____
24._____	Great desire for sweet foods	24._____
25._____	Bad breath	25._____
26._____	Subject to colds and infection	26._____
27._____	Require tranquilizers	27._____
28._____	Use pep pills	28._____

29.___	Use antacids	29. _____
30.___	Have that "blah" feeling	30. _____
31.___	Other symptom	31. _____
32.___	Other symptom	32. _____

My program includes pure, potent nutritional supplements and not drugs. They provide a balanced nutrient base enabling the body to heal many unhealthy conditions. To experience perfect health we must provide perfect nutritional intake. We must also provide other perfect health experiences too, such as perfect exercise and perfect rest. However, unfortunately, no program is perfect so we will never be perfect. However, we can be much better than we are.

For more information contact:
C J Buchanan & Companies
info@cjbuchanan.com **or** www.ask4clive.com
Phone: 435-275-6649

Chapter 1
The Beginning

I have been asked many times to explain how I overcame MS and what herbs I use to do so. It should be pointed out, I still have MS but MS does not have me.

I was a very sickly child and caught everything that came to town. I had severe allergies, asthma, and reoccurring pneumonia. I was physically strong, I wrestled, played football, and participated in many extracurricular activities in school, but constant illness stopped me from achieving much of what I desired.

About age 23, I started having strange maladies. When my leg dragged, the doctor always blamed it on the bullet that was in my leg from an accident in my youth. When I had double vision, the doctor blamed it on the explosion and glass in my eyes that left me blind for a couple of weeks. When I became tired and fatigued when I got overheated, the doctor blamed it on the family ticker. Our family has a history of heart and cardiovascular conditions. My mother died of a heart condition when she was 43 and my father died of a heart attack at the age of 48.

The explanations for my symptoms were so good, neither my doctors nor I thought to look for another cause. I had symptoms for over 17 years before I was diagnosed with Multiple Sclerosis (MS).

One day, in 1984, I happened on a book about chlorine and heart disease. It presented excellent documentation that chlorinated drinking water increases your chance of a heart attack.

I started doing research on water filters. During my studies, I stumbled on an article titled "Bee Pollen: The Miracle Food". It said Bee Pollen helped allergies. As a long time allergy sufferer, that got my attention so I read the article. It claimed that Bee Pollen helped almost everything. In fact, it said Bee Pollen would do so much that I did not believe it. I almost didn't try it. Lucky for me, I did try it. My allergies improved. My asthma mostly went away. Best of all, all my strange maladies disappeared.

Then a (hopefully well meaning) doctor told me Bee Pollen may be good for other people, but it was poisoning my system. He said I should stop taking it. Like a dummy I did. Have you ever followed the advice of an expert and found out that it was wrong? My allergies came back, my asthma came back, and

I had a disabling MS attack that left me unable to write, walk, or speak, without slurring. I had some use of my arms and legs, but no feeling. I could crawl, but very slowly.

I went to a new doctor. He immediately recognized that most of my problems were symptoms of MS. He ran tests for cancer, tumors, strokes and other conditions, in addition to the ones for MS. Six weeks later, when I got the confirmation that I had MS I was relieved. It was good to know it was not all in my head. I asked the doctor for a prognosis. Based on my history of relapsing remitting symptoms followed by a consistent increase in symptoms he thought I had secondary progressive MS. He said my condition would slowly deteriorate. His prediction was grim at best.

A few weeks later, an old friend came to visit me. When she saw my condition she was shocked. My speech was so slurred she had trouble understanding me. My arms, legs and head were shaking non-stop. It was so dismaying for her to see a close friend in this condition that she could not bring herself to come to my side of the room.

When my friend left I was determined I would walk again. I got the doctor on the phone and demanded a cure. After a long argument he said, "Clive you must accept the fact that you are going to spend the rest of your life watching TV with someone else changing the channels." That made me all the more determined to walk.

Later that day, when I was all alone, I forced myself to my feet and attempted to walk. As my body began to move forward I realized my feet were not moving. I tried to bring my arms forward to break my fall, but they did not move fast enough. I fell hard on my face. Strange as it seems, it may have been the best day of my life.

There, on the floor, somewhat dazed, it was like I saw a vision. I saw myself standing in front of huge audiences, teaching that in this life it does not matter what happens to you. It matters how you respond to it. You might not control everything or everyone around you, but you do control how you respond. I taught that everyone has a condition or trial that is the equivalent of my MS.

A curtain dropped and opened and I began to teach a new message. You must take responsibility for your own life. You should not blame anyone else for your problems. Get the best information you can find and then make your own decisions. If you do not like something either change it or change your attitude.

Finally, I began extolling the virtues of holistic health. I was teaching about herbs, food supplements, success, and leadership. You and thousands like you were there in my vision. At that instant in time, over thirty years ago, my whole life changed forever.

As I came to myself, my mind was flooded with ideas of mental games, supplements, and exercises that would help me overcome MS. The product that first came to me was a high quality Bee Pollen. It seemed more important than all the other supplements. If Transfer Factor had been available I think it would have been number one.

I called my new doctor and asked if Bee Pollen could have made my MS worse. He told me no. I asked him if Bee Pollen could help the condition. He said he didn't know, but that it would not hurt. I put down the telephone and crawled into the kitchen. My wife gave me a teaspoon of Bee Pollen. I sat there by the refrigerator for a couple of hours, and then took a second teaspoon of Bee Pollen. I waited another two hours and took a third teaspoon of Bee Pollen. (One teaspoon is the amount recommended for most people.)
Six hours later I was walking again. I was not walking well and leaning heavily on a walking stick, but I was walking. (I do not recommend anyone who has not previously taken Bee Pollen start with three teaspoons. That much Bee Pollen would detoxify the systems of most people too rapidly and could make the person very ill. Follow the instructions on the bottle)

From that day to this with few exceptions, I take at least three teaspoons of Bee Pollen a day. In fighting Multiple Sclerosis the first and most important product was Bee Pollen. Today, it is a tossup between Bee Pollen and Transfer Factor. If I had allergies, I would start out with one granule of Bee Pollen a day. Take this amount for one week. Then I would increase to two granules a day for a week, then four granules a day for a week, eight granules a day for a week. Then an eighth of a teaspoon everyday for a week is about right. Then from that point on, I would increase by an eighth of a teaspoon each week until I was eventually taking three teaspoons of Bee Pollen a day (One teaspoon before each meal). I should point out there is a big difference in Bee Pollens. My instructions are for the best of Pollens.

If at any time, I found my allergies getting worse, I would reduce the amount of Bee Pollen that I was taking by three fourths. I would take that amount for a full month before trying to increase again.

If I did not have allergies, I would start with an eighth of a teaspoon of Bee Pollen each day for a week. I would increase each week by an eighth of a teaspoon until I reached one teaspoon of Bee Pollen before each meal.

I find that taking this amount of Bee Pollen gives me increased energy. I do not have the fatigue normally associated with Multiple Sclerosis. And my exacerbation's "attacks", if any, are very infrequent and so mild I am unaware of them.

There is a relatively new product that was not available when I first struggled with MS. It is called Transfer Factor. I would take it in its classic form. This product educates your immune system. It is the only product that makes your immune system smarter. It teaches your body not to attack itself. It also helps your body recognize and destroy invading organisms. I have met people who claim to have overcome all their MS symptoms using this product alone. When I first started research on this product I was so impressed I wrote a book on it. The name of the book is Transfer Factor Against Inhuman Terrorists.

If I were to have an MS attack, I would immediately begin taking Evening Primrose Oil at the rate of six capsules a day. If Evening Primrose Oil were not available, I would take Black Currant Oil, Borage Oil, or Flaxseed Oil. I would only take this product during exacerbations.

The reason I would only take Evening Primrose Oil during an attack is because it reduces inflammation and excessive auto immune response, but if taken all the time the body gets used to it. Then it stops working. It will not help you when you really need it. To get the full power of Evening Primrose Oil use it with discretion.

To help me rebuild my nerves I would take Classic Transfer Factor, Bee Pollen, a B-Complex or a multivitamin high in the B vitamins and the herb, Gotu Kola. To help my body deal with fat more efficiently I would take Lecithin. To help me rebuild my muscles I would take L-Carnitine. For additional energy I would take Siberian Ginseng. To keep my body cool I would drink plenty of liquids.

Products and their amounts:

Bee Pollen - 3 teaspoons a day -- 1 teaspoon before each meal. (Remember to work up on the Pollen very slowly).

Classic Transfer Factor 9 capsules per day. This can be reduced to 3 after a year.

Multivitamin with a high B-Complex – As directed.

Lecithin - three 400mg capsules a day or one 1200mg capsule a day.

Gotu Kola - 3 capsules a day -- 1 capsule before each meal.

L-Carnitine - 500mg per day.

Siberian Ginseng - 3 capsules a day.

Evening Primrose Oil - 2 capsules three times a day. (Only when experiencing an exacerbation.)

Chapter 2
Do's, Do Not's, and Check Out's

Do: Exercise (at a moderate level so that you do not overheat yourself) for at least thirty minutes six days a week. I would work towards a goal of at least forty-five minutes a day. If the only exercise that you can do is crawl, then start with crawling.

Studies done at the University of Utah suggest that exercising forty-five minutes a day greatly reduces the frequency of MS exacerbations. It could reduce them more than any of the drugs currently on the market. The studies also show faster remissions in those with relapsing, remitting MS.

More recently studies by MS. Doctors Bombardier and Bowen suggest that aerobic exercise is a better treatment for depression than standard antidepressant medication. Seems it has a more effective longer lasting effect than the drugs. It also has a much lower incidence of side effects.

Do: Believe you can get well. I know you have been told that MS is an incurable progressive condition. The truth is there are no incurable conditions only incurable people. We have not found all the cures, but we will. The remedy may require more work and belief than you have. Only you know if or how soon you will give up. I hope you never stop looking for a way to get better. You must believe and keep working, seeking, and trying if you are to have any hope of improving. Remember even false hope is better than no hope at all.

Do: Believe that God is a just God and that hidden somewhere in every challenge there is a blessing greater than the challenge.

Do: Play mind games that teach your subconscious mind what you want it to do. It can give instructions to every part of your body. I am a science fiction fan. Some of the tools I use in my mind game do not exist yet. In my fantasy (mind game) I am in a miniature hovercraft floating over my brain. I am inspecting the myelin for holes. When I see a hole I zoom in on it. There I see grubby little men with picks and shovels chopping away at my myelin sheath. With a loud speaker I tell them to stop. They never do so I shoot them with a ray gun. Then I have a tool that sprays liquid myelin. I use it to fill the hole then I move on looking for another hole. When all the holes are found and filled I stop playing the game for a day. You can make up your own game. Just be sure it is visually graphic to your subconscious mind and the damage to the myelin is both stopped and repaired.

Do not under estimate the power of the subconscious mind. In a study done at Harvard University students were given caffeine tablets and told that they were sleeping pills. A full half the students in the study reported sleeping better after taking the pill. Some aborigine medicine men tell healthy members of their tribe that they will die on a specific day and they do.

Do: Get plenty of sunshine. It has long been known that people who lived in warm climates were less likely to get MS. Why has been a mystery. Recently studies have linked low Vitamin D levels to exacerbations. This may also explain why a high percentage of MS victims are overachievers. They often spend more time indoors working. It would be better if they were out in the sunshine soaking up Vitamin D.

Do: Remove cheese from your diet. Cheese, an otherwise good food is like poison to people with Multiple Sclerosis. Most Cheese contains tyramine, an amino that is formed in the ageing or fermenting of some foods and beverages. It has a very negative effect on most people with MS. It often causes intense headaches for some people on MAOI inhibitors.

Do not drink: All alcoholic beverages impair brain function and should be avoided by anyone with MS. Red wine has a large amount of tyramine and much like cheese should always be avoided. Tyramine is found in most if not all alcoholic beverages. Some believe it is the main cause of hangovers.

Check Out: Some scholars suggest you restrict or totally eliminate gluten from the diet. It has been my experience that some do better without gluten and others do just as well with gluten. You need to experiment.

Check Out: There was a time when doctors and herbalists thought chocolate was bad for everyone. Today we have learned that a little chocolate is good for almost everyone. Dark Chocolate is the best for you. Most people with MS can safely enjoy it but it does have a little tyramine and some do better if they eliminate chocolate.

Chapter 3
Bee Pollen

Records of the use of Pollen date back 15,000 years. At Cuevas de la Arana, near Bicorp, Valencia, Spain, prehistoric cave paintings depicting men foraging for Honey and Pollen were discovered in 1919. One painting depicts a man climbing a rope to a hole in a cliff where he takes a honeycomb and puts it in some type of a container. Beekeeping scenes from at least four ancient Egyptian tombs have been photographed and may be seen in the Metropolitan Museum of Art in New York City. The bees and hives are easily recognizable with identical hives that are still in use today in undeveloped parts of Africa.

Until about 1960, pure Pollen could not be obtained directly from the hive. The honeybees deposited it immediately into a honeycomb and added nectar.

This blend of Honey and Pollen is called Bee Bread by modern day beekeepers. Prior to about 200 years ago it was called honey. About 1960 (It may have been invented before but not patented) a method of collecting Pollen was invented which forces the bees to crawl through a narrow mesh screen before they enter the hive. Pollen pellets or pods are brushed off their loaded hind legs as they enter into the hive. The Pollen pods drop through another screen with smaller holes into a collection drawer. If the Pollen is gathered from a variety of plants, the pollen will be multicolored. The color of the Pollen will be uniform if the hive is placed in an area with a single flower such as a large field of clover. The color of the Pollen has nothing to do with the virtues of Pollen as a food. It does indicate the variety of flowers from which the bees collected. Once the Pollen pods have fallen into the collection drawer, they are retrieved, dried, cleaned and stored. The collection, cleaning and stabilization of Pollen should be performed in a manner so as not to compromise the nutrient or enzyme content of the Pollen.

Pollen consists of myriads of microspores formed in the anthers of flowering plants, and in the staminate cones of conifers and cycads. The individual Pollen spores are very small. A single strobilus may produce six million pollen grains. Many plants are pollinated by wind. Water currents are responsible for pollinating other plants, and still others may be pollinated by rain. These are the pollens most people are allergic to. Bees do not collect Pollen from these plants. They gather sticky Pollen usually found in showy or scented flowers with nectar. The plants with this type flower are largely insect pollinated. Insect pollinators include flies, beetles, bugs, wasps, bees, butterflies and moths. Hummingbirds, sunbirds and other nectar eating pollinators also participate in the pollination process.

Pollen is a complete food and is in a form easily assimilated by the body. It is known to regulate and stimulate metabolism by supplying the missing factors that may not be supplied in other foods.

Many scientific studies have and are currently being done on the benefits of Pollen. Various clinics are and have been experimenting with Pollen in relation to many ailments. Questions like: How does Pollen speed healing after an injury? Can Pollen be used as a sole source of nutrients for prolonged periods? And how does Pollen increase energy?

Paavo Airola, N.D., Ph.D., had this to say, "Pollen is the richest and most complete food in nature. It increases the body's resistance to stress and disease and also speeds up the healing process in most conditions of ill health; Pollen also possesses age-retarding and rejuvenating properties. Truly, Bee Pollen is a miracle food, a wonder medicine and a true Fountain of Youth."

RAW BEE POLLEN WEIGHT BREAKDOWN*

454,000mg. per pound
28,000mg. per ounce
14,000mg. per tablespoon
4,700mg. per teaspoon
3,575mg. per ¾ teaspoon
2,383mg. per ½ teaspoon
1,192mg. per ¼ teaspoon
596mg per 1/8 teaspoon

*These figures are based upon weight and not volume. This table is designed to aid those who wish to switch over to raw Bee Pollen granules from Bee Pollen tablets/capsules, and is only to be used as an approximate comparison.

Pollen tablets and capsules are convenient but usually have lower nutrient and enzyme content. In many cases the Pollen used in tablets and capsules is of lower quality even before it is processed. I am not a big fan of so called Potentized Pollen because it removes a natural coating which keeps the Pollen potent. When this coating is removed the Pollen becomes rancid very quickly. Heat, moisture, and chemicals are all enemies of Bee Pollen and reduce its potency. Pollen retains its potency best when it is air dried and vacuum packed. Once a container is opened it should be stored in a frost free refrigerator.

Chapter 4
Transfer Factor

Transfer Factor is a molecule that acts like an educator that teaches your immune system to discern what it should and should not attack. It works like a cross between a college professor and a pep squad educating and encouraging greater effort from our white blood cells and other body defense systems. There are hundreds of different transfer factors. In this book these factors, as a group, will be called Transfer Factor.

Harmful viruses, parasites, fungi, mold, and bacteria disguise themselves as benign residents of the body. The human body is well prepared and ready to handle most invaders but only if it can distinguish which invaders are harmful and which are friendly.

Transfer Factor helps the body know the good from the bad. Dr. William J. Hennen, Ph.D. in his book Natural Immune Booster Transfer Factor explains Transfer Factor this way, "Transfer Factors are small immune messenger molecules that are produced by higher organisms. Their role is to transfer immune recognition signals between immune cells and thereby assist in educating naïve immune cells about a present or potential danger."

Transfer Factor was first discovered way back in 1949, but only recently became commercially available. Transfer Factor cannot be synthesized; it must be extracted from white blood cells, Colostrum or Egg Yokes. It took decades and millions of dollars to discover how to harvest it.

Why was the uncovering of Transfer Factor not heralded as the greatest discovery of all time? Because, it came at a time when many new antibiotics were being discovered. History may well call this time the beginning of the antibiotic age. Researchers of the time believed that by the year 2000 all infectious disease would be wiped out.

Finding and isolating Transfer Factors was a more complex challenge than finding and isolating a single chemical like those found in most standard pharmaceutical drugs.

Since Transfer Factor's discovery in 1949 an estimated $40,000,000 has been spent on research.

In excess of 3,000 scientific papers have been published extolling the virtues of these tiny molecules.

Transfer Factor has more than one roll to play in the fight against MS. Earlier we talked about how it teaches the body not to attack itself. Studies show that whenever someone with MS has a fever the MS symptoms temporarily get worse. Every time you avoid a cold, flu, or other illness you will likely avoid a fever. That means fewer MS symptoms.

It is commonly believed that exacerbations often follow illnesses. This may be because the immune system is operating at a higher level but does not know what to attack after the cold or flu has been defeated. Another possibility is the increased stress caused by illness. Many believe both symptoms and exacerbations increase with stress. In any case, being well mentally, spiritually, or physically slows the progression of Multiple Sclerosis.

To learn more about Transfer Factor get my book Transfer Factor Against Inhuman Terrorists.

You will have good days and bad days. Get the best out of the good days. The best advice I was given by a friend with MS was,

"Take pie when pie is offered!"

Chapter 5
Lecithin

What is Lecithin? In chemical terms, Lecithin is known as a phospholipid. This means it is composed of a combination of fatty acids, phosphorus, and nitrogen. In the body, phospholipids are used to transport fats. Phospholipids are an important constituent of the lipoproteins that are needed to carry cholesterol safely through the blood stream. In their absence, serious abnormalities of fat transport can occur.

Lecithin and cholesterol are found in every cell of the body. Phospholipids and cholesterol are present in both the cell membrane and in the membranes of the tiny internal organelles in the cell. Both cholesterol and the phospholipids have controlling effects on the permeability of cell membranes. This is because these are some of the few substances, which are not soluble in water. Hence the structure of the cell membranes is held together mainly by phospholipids (like Lecithin), and cholesterol.

Lecithin is composed of Phosphoric Acid, Choline and Inositol. It is well established that Phosphoric Acid forms part of all bones and is high in nerve and brain tissue. It also forms part of the Adenosine-Triphosphate that furnishes energy for many of the cell reactions of the body.

Choline forms part of the acetylcholine in the brain. This substance is a neurotransmitter meaning it is necessary for the brain cells to communicate with one another. This fact has given rise to the notion that Lecithin is good food for the brain.

Choline deficiency causes cholesterol and blood pressure levels to rise. On the other hand, a high Choline diet enables the blood cells to last longer, causing an increased hemoglobin count. This in turn brings more oxygen to the tissues, stimulating greater cell activity and cell replication.

Choline is important for the syntheses of nucleic acid in the center of every cell, and also for the production of DNA and RNA, factors on heredity. It aids Lecithin in the conversion of fats on the liver. Choline deficiencies also produce muscular dystrophy and "fatty liver disease."

Inositol, the third component of Lecithin, is ten times more prevalent in the body than any other vitamin, except Niacin. Inositol affects fat metabolism. Deficiencies in Inositol result in loss of hair, constipation, eczema, eye disorders, reproductive failure, and growth abnormalities. Like Choline, Inositol reduces the amount of cholesterol in the blood.

Since Phosphoric Acid, Choline, and Inositol are so vital in so many functions, it is important to maintain a high level in the body.

The more animal fats you eat, the more conscientious you should be about the amount of Lecithin you take. Why? Animal fats have the highest percentage of cholesterol; and Lecithin acts to dissolve cholesterol.
Lecithin is necessary to every cell and organ in the body as it is found in every cell and organ. Organs can be helped and rebuilt by eating Lecithin in sufficient amounts. Once repaired, Lecithin helps to maintain these organs. It has been surmised that a deficiency of Lecithin in the diet may be one of the causes of aging.

Improvements that can be traced to the addition of Lecithin to the diet are: A better memory, healthier skin, and sounder mental and nerve status. Lecithin is also fundamental in the absorption and digestion of vitamin A, D, E, and K.

The most common benefits attributed to Lecithin are: improved nerve health, less nervous exhaustion, better processing of fat and cholesterol, better brain function, lower blood pressure, increased gamma globulin in the blood, improved infection resistance, fewer skin disturbances such as eczema, acne, and psoriasis, and softening of aging skin.

Chapter 6
Gotu Kola

Gotu Kola is considered a prime nerve tonic in Ayurvedic medicine to promote mental clarity, and is used to treat stress, nervousness and many nervous system disorders, according to Planetary Herbology by Michael Tierra, C.A., ND. Many people confuse Gotu Kola with Kola, a caffeine-containing herb. However, The Honest New Herbal by Varro Tyler, Ph.D., reports Gotu Kola's effects are not due to caffeine but to glycosides, which have shown mild sedative effects in animals.

There are many theories why memories become lost or concentration begins to falter as we age. Until recently, amino acids, vitamins and minerals have traditionally received the brunt of the attention given to nutritional and cerebral function. But as the popularity of herbs rises, all that is changing. Retailers are seeing skyrocketing sales of botanicals such as Gotu Kola and Ginkgo Biloba, and a host of other herbs said to influence brain function.

Natural supplements are just now being considered by main stream doctors, however when studies are done the results are usually good. Ginkgo Biloba was studied at the MS Center of Oregon to see if it would help attention span. The results showed measurable improvement when compared with an inactive placebo. As good as Ginkgo is I like Gotu Kola better. It appears to me to help a wider verity of conditions.

The brain relies on a constant stream of blood sugar, nutrients and oxygen to produce the energy used to direct our every thought and action. Each brain cell, or neuron, manufactures neurotransmitters, chemical substances that allow the neurons to communicate with each other. All memory, learning, thoughts, actions and emotions depend on the neuron's ability to make them.

Thousands of tiny capillaries transport oxygen-rich red blood cells to the neurons. However, the Optimal Nutritional Review newsletter reports that as we age, arteriosclerosis can slowly constrict the capillaries and reduce cerebral blood flow. Without an adequate blood supply, the cells become starved for nutrients and oxygen, and malfunctions such as memory loss, personality changes and inability to concentrate or communicate can result.

Research also shows that excess fats and toxic free radicals combine in the bloodstream, causing brain cells to produce lipofuscin, a waste product of brain metabolism.

Gerontologists believe lipofuscin, which can fill up to 75 percent of the neuronic volume in the elderly, disrupts the cell's function and may even kill it, according to Brainfood: Nutrition and Your Brain by Brian and Roberta Morgan.

Historically, Gotu Kola is considered one of the best herbal nerve tonics. Because Gotu Kola acts as a cleanser of the blood, it follows that it strengthens the heart, balances the hormones and the nervous system. As a result of improving blood circulation Gotu Kola is good when used after a nervous breakdown. It is able to rebuild energy reserves. For this reason, it is called 'food for the brain'. It increases mental and physical power. It combats stress and improves reflexes. Gotu Kola has an energizing effect on the cells of the brain. It relieves high blood pressure, mental fatigue, and senility, and helps the body defend itself against various toxins.

Gotu Kola contains vitamins A, G (Riboflavin Complex, also known as vitamin B_2), and K and is high in Magnesium. Kate McCann, C.N., nutritionist and supplements buyer for Vitality Unlimited in Santa Fe, NM., says Gotu Kola and Ginkgo are the two most popular herbs in the store for brain function. "People definitely come in looking and asking for them, and sales really pick up during the final exam time of the school year," she says. McCann notes that Gotu Kola customers say it helps them avoid mental fatigue during long work hours.

Gotu Kola is known as the memory herb because it is known to stimulate circulation. It is valued as a nervous system restorative, used to combat fatigue, and to improve memory. It is the favorite food of Elephants and you know what they say about elephants. (They never forget!) It is one of the key ingredients in a product called Transfer Factor Recall. Transfer Factor Recall is the best brain support product I have ever seen.

Chapter 7
L-Carnitine

L-Carnitine was discovered in 1905. It has been scrutinized in over 2,000 scientific studies, and is used successfully to treat seriously ill patients of all ages.

Carnitine is not an essential amino acid because the liver can manufacture it. Generally just referred to as an amino, it is a protein-like nutrient manufactured in the body and available in foods. However, it is so important in providing energy to muscles, including the heart, that some researchers are now recommending Carnitine supplements in the diet.

In 1959, I. B. Fritz discovered that when Carnitine from muscle is added to liver tissue, it increases the rate at which the liver oxidizes fats, thereby increasing the amount of energy available. It was found that Carnitine acts by carrying fat across a membrane into the energy-burning mitochondria of each cell. The more Carnitine available, the faster fat is transported and the more fat is oxidized for energy. This energy is then stored not as fat, but as Adenosine Triphosphate (ATP), the trigger for many of the body's activities, including muscle contraction. Thus, Carnitine's primary role seems to be to regulate fat metabolism. If Carnitine is absent or deficient, long-chain fatty acids cannot be burned efficiently; they will then tend to build up in and around the cell and in the bloodstream as fats and triglycerides.

Carnitine does increase the rate in which fat is burned, and also makes it possible to exercise longer without fatigue. This may make it easier for those who want to improve their chances of losing weight by exercising.

Carnitine has another function directly related to energy availability. It helps the body to oxidize amino acids when necessary. Amino acids are not a primary source of energy but when a person exercises for a long time, the limited carbohydrate stored in the muscles may all be used up, and fat may not be immediately available. Or when someone fasts (whether deliberately or involuntarily, as during famine), the muscles may begin to consume branched-chain amino acids for fuel. Carnitine may make this substitution possible.

Carnitine may also have some involvement in prostaglandin metabolism. Prostaglandins contribute to the functioning of smooth muscle. Thus, Carnitine may be crucial for all the muscles of the body: It regulates fat burning in the heart (whose main source of energy may be fat) and in skeletal muscles; it helps to change branched-chain amino acids into fuel for the skeletal muscles when necessary; and it plays some role in prostaglandin metabolism in smooth muscles.

The location of Carnitine in the body has given researchers clues about its functions and, therefore, possible clinical uses. It is most highly concentrated in the heart (particularly the sarcoplasmic reticulum), the organ to which fat oxidation is most crucial for energy. In fact, the heart contains more Carnitine than any other organ, and some of Carnitine's most important clinical applications are in heart disease.

Carnitine is involved in many of the body's metabolic processes. Besides controlling blood sugar and protein metabolism, Carnitine is involved in transporting signals between cells and the brain, in reducing blood serum cholesterol and triglycerides, in boosting endurance for stress, in improving pulse recovery rate following exercise, and in utilizing fats more efficiently so that they do not build up in the system.

Although the brain depends exclusively on glucose for energy, Carnitine is also found there, especially in the cerebellum. Its role in the brain remains to be discovered, however it has been shown to improve brain function.

Deficiencies of Carnitine are found in certain genetic abnormalities and in several neuromuscular disorders. Systemic Carnitine deficiency can lead to acidic blood, brain degeneration like that in Reye's syndrome and progressive muscle weakness.

Carnitine therapy may also be useful in a wide variety of clinical conditions. Carnitine supplementation may be worth a try in any form of hyperlipidemia or muscle weakness. Athletes, particularly in Europe, use Carnitine supplements for improved endurance. Carnitine may improve muscle building by improving fat utilization and is often useful in treating obesity.

Chapter 8
Siberian Ginseng

Herbalists have traditionally thought of Ginseng as a "tonic," an herb taken over an extended period of time for its cumulative effects of nourishing and strengthening the body. In particular, Ginseng affects the glandular tissues such as the adrenal and endocrine glands, which regulate many body functions. In 1958, Russian scientists concluded that Ginseng is an "adaptogen," a substance that helps the whole body adapt to physical and mental strain.

Whatever term is used, tonic or adaptogen, traditional use and scientific research come to the same conclusion: Ginseng is an herb that affects the whole body. Both research and clinical use have confirmed the herb's anti-aging affects and its ability to normalize blood pressure, boost the immune system, reduce cholesterol and stimulate mental activity. It can also normalize blood sugar levels in diabetics, improve vision and hearing, strengthen the nervous system and stimulate various endocrine functions, including sexual energy.

More recent research indicates that Ginseng can enhance the affect of cancer-fighting drugs and improve pulmonary functions. The latest research also confirms the claim that Ginseng can help overcome the strain of exercise on the heart and lungs.

Even though Ginseng obviously can benefit health problems, American herbalists suggest Ginseng more often for its overall effects than for its ability to treat specific ailments. Michael Tierra, a doctor of Oriental medicine in Santa Cruz, CA, often suggests Ginseng when lack of energy or weakness of digestion is a symptom.

In the Orient, Ginseng is called the King of Herbs. It stimulates the entire body energy to overcome stress, fatigue and weakness. It is especially stimulating for mental fatigue. It stimulates and improves brain cell functions. Ginseng has a very beneficial effect on the heart and circulation. It is considered by many to be a cure-all herb. It acts as an antidote to various types of drugs and toxic chemicals and it is said to protect the body against radiation. It is said to improve vision and hearing activity, improve working ability, and help to reduce irritability. Some take it to gain poise and composure.

Even as I write this book studies are going on at the MS Center in Portland to see how much it improves mental alertness and reduces fatigue.

Ginseng contains vitamins A and E. It also contains Thiamin, Riboflavin, B12, Niacin, Calcium, Iron, Phosphorus, Sodium, Silicon, Potassium, Manganese, Sulfur and Tin.

Remember the world is a better place because you are here.

You have the power to make it so.

Chapter 9
Evening Primrose Oil

The Evening Primrose is a gorgeous yellow flower. Its petals open at twilight and close at the crack of dawn early in the season. Later on, as the summer wears on, the flowers stay open all day long.

All parts of the plant can be used. The root is often boiled and tastes very much like a sweet parsnip. Sometimes the roots are pickled and used in tossed salads. The leaf and stems of the plant can be used to make a tea which will soothe a cough.

Evening Primrose is best known for its oil which is squeezed from the seeds. The oil contains Gamma Linolic Acid, often referred to as GLA. This substance balances the immune system and helps to prevent overreaction. Evening Primrose Oil is often used as a cure for a hangover. It takes approximately five capsules to get rid of the hangover.

Evening Primrose Oil stops MS exacerbations because it reduces inflammation. It works like a natural steroid without the side effects associated with synthetic steroids. It also eases menopausal discomfort and aids in PMS. In fact, in the herbal world, Evening Primrose Oil is best known for its benefits in treating PMS. Louise Tenney, in her book, Health Handbook, said it will help alcoholism, allergies, asthma, arthritis, glaucoma, headaches, heart disease, menstruation, PMS, lower cholesterol, obesity, reduces blood pressure, helps skin and hair health, aids in eczema and reduces hyperactivity in children. It is a powerful herb even though very little is written about it.

Chapter 10
It's All Up to You

If you have read this book up to this point with an open mind you will likely find a way to be free of many if not all your MS symptoms. I cannot promise that if you follow this system you will completely overcome MS. I wish I could. I can promise that if you follow this system you will be healthier than you would have been otherwise. I can say this with confidence because good nutrition and proper thinking is beneficial for everyone.

The three most important things to remember are:

1. In this life it does not matter what happens to you, it matters how you respond to it. Within every challenge there is a blessing greater than the challenge. The way you chose to respond will determine whether or not you find and receive the blessing.

2. Take responsibility for your own life. Do not blame anyone or anything else for your problems. Do not give credit to anyone for that which you have achieved. Do acknowledge those who have helped you on your way. When it comes to your health get the best advice from the most knowledgeable people you can find, but make your own decisions. Do not let any doctor, family member, friend, naturopath, or herbalist bully you into doing something you do not feel good about.

3. If you choose to follow this program follow it completely. If you are driving a car you must make sure it has engine coolant, brake fluid, oil, transmission fluid, and gasoline. If you leave out any one of these necessities the car will not run very long. If you follow only part of the program you will only get part of the benefit. Because the parts of the program work synergistically if you only follow one half the program you will only get about one forth the results.

Some people wallow in their misfortune and have on going pity parties. They feel so sorry for themselves that they live their lives in misery and make other people do for them what they should be doing for themselves. This is a luxury you cannot afford. Do everything you can for yourself. Enjoy what you can do and give thanks that you can do it. (Yes I know that's easy advice to give and harder to follow. Remember I have been there.)

Another great bit of advice that a friend gave me when I was first diagnosed, "Take pie when pie is offered." Meaning, enjoy your good days and every good thing that is offered. Enjoy life and prosper.

The Multiple Sclerosis Society is a great source of support. It lets you know you are not alone.

They are working hard but they do not have all the answers.

Learn from many sources and make up your own mind in what you do.

You are the boss!

Chapter 11
It's Good to Know

This is not part of the program but knowing it will make your life better. When the diagnosis of Multiple Sclerosis is first received most people will either be relieved that it is not something worse like ALS or they go into shock. When the knowledge sinks in there is almost always a period of shock. Then comes denial. The doctor can't be right. And finally depression sets in. Depression is fed by fear. When you never know what the next day will bring fear is natural. If you have been through these steps it only means you are normal.

All these steps are hard on the family emotionally. Some people are not strong enough to live with someone with MS. Divorce rates are high. This sounds discouraging. But it does not have to be. Like everything else in life it is a state of mind. There are healthy millionaires who should be filled with joy and thanks giving who are so sad and depressed they commit suicide. There are sick people living in cardboard shacks who are happy and joyful. It is all a state of mind. When your spouse sticks with you and supports you that is wonderful. You know you are living with a great person. If your spouse is weak and leaves that is good too because now you are free to find someone good enough to deserve you. It is all attitude. The one thing you will always control is the way you think.

I met a man yesterday wearing a neck brace because of MS. He said MS was a new beginning. He was now finding joy in life he would never have found had it not been for MS. MS helps you find out who you are. You discover who your real friends are. Every day is a new adventure as you learn how to cope with new challenges. It saved me from a life of drudgery working at a job I really did not like.

I believe the two greatest challenges of MS are the fear and the discouragement/depression. Fear comes from worrying about the future and what might happen tomorrow. Remember the section on the mind games. Think about tomorrow being the way you want it to be given your current circumstances. You really do tend to get what you think about, good or bad. If you only think of the good you will get more of it.

Depression and discouragement come from thinking about the past and that life is not fair. You think your life should be better so you either develop a victim or a blame mentality. You blame someone or something (usually MS) for everything. It is very easy to blame everything that happens on either someone who did not stand by you or MS. The truth is we all have equal challenges; they just come in different packages.

The secret is to live in the present. Think about what you can do not what you can't do. With all the developments to help deal with symptoms you will have a very near normal life expectancy. People with MS as a group have higher incomes than the population as a whole. They tend to be over-achievers. They have a much greater appreciation of the little things. Before MS I had no appreciation of walking. Having once lost the ability to walk, walking now brings me great joy. Night and peripheral vision were not even acknowledged till they disappeared. When they came back they were gifts from God. You can be happy.

People with Multiple Sclerosis need money too. Fortunately, most people with MS are able to keep their jobs and labor laws are meant to prevent discrimination. Some professions simply cannot be done by someone with MS. Can you picture a dentist with either a numb or shaky hand? Despite the labor laws discrimination exists when you are looking for a new job or a promotion. On the face of it this discrimination seems like a bad thing. In truth, it may be the very reason people with MS earn above average incomes.

You can start a home based business. There are wide varieties of things you can do from home. The three businesses that earn people the most money are internet, real-estate, and network marketing businesses. All of these are easy if you: 1. have a system, 2. have someone to teach you the system, and 3. the patience and willingness to learn and work the system.

When I first recovered the ability to walk and talk so I could be easily understood no one would employ me doing anything except some charity type minimum wage jobs. The only option I was aware of at the time was network marketing. (Also known as MLM, direct marketing, and POD. Not to be confused with pyramid schemes.) It took me about a year to get my income up to that of my peers in my graduating class. In two years I was earning more than most of them. Why I gave it up to become a speaker and a writer I cannot say. I guess it may have been ego. Recently I realized MLM was a great profession that I truly enjoyed. So I researched the companies currently available to join and began working with a company that fit me. The real beauty of network marketing is that it provides residual income in addition to the current checks.

Women with MS often ask, "Is it safe for me to get pregnant?" Tending children when you have MS is not always easy. I would consult my physician. MS is not an inherited disease. You cannot pass it on to your children. According to Inside MS the official magazine of the National Multiple Sclerosis Society, "Research points toward infections rather than something toxic in air, water or food as a triggering agent, though recent evidence hints that a lack of sun exposure, leading to lower vitamin D levels, may play a role." A susceptibility to MS may be inherited. Being pregnant seems to protect against exacerbations. The frequency and duration of events are reduced. It is believed to be hormone related.

Stay active. Do not hibernate. Life is full of fun enlightening things you can do. I enjoy cruising. Most modern cruise ships are wheelchair friendly. They have cabins to facilitate those with challenges. I take groups on cruises once or twice a year. We have wonderful empowering seminars on the days we are at sea and most people in the group get a tax write off. Feel free to contact me next time you are feeling like an ocean voyage.

Find a worthy cause you can help. Help a good person get elected. Support a missionary, volunteer to help your favorite charity, the list of possibilities is endless. The more you are involved outside of you the less you will worry and many of your problems will either just go away or seem not so bad.

Stay cool but not cold on the inside. Either hot or cold can make symptoms worse. Try to keep yourself well hydrated. Always be sipping on a cool drink. Water is the best. Avoid diet drinks. One of the most common artificial sweeteners, Aspartame has been linked to symptoms much like MS. Recent studies link it to cancer. I stress AVOID ASPARTAME! Sometimes all the liquid drinking means an extra stop at the restroom but it is worth it to live more like the rest of the world.

Track your efforts to follow the program. In business there is a saying, "That which is measured improves." During times when money is tight, symptoms are worse or when symptoms are gone it is easy to let some or all of the program slide. This is true even after it is a habit. I have received many e-mails or phone calls from people who got off the program, thinking they didn't need it anymore or that it was not working. After about six months they are ready to get back on the program.

I have included an evaluation sheet to help you track your improvement. I put it at the first so you would not miss it. The reports in the back are to help you stay on track. There is a six week supply. Feel free to copy the reports when you run out.

You are unique. There is no one just like you. There are many who face similar challenges. You can be a victor and change MS from a curse to a blessing. (Even though it may not seem like a blessing today.)

I cannot predict your future because you and God are in control. You may just slow down the progression of the condition. You may get total remission. All I can promise is that if you follow the program you will be in better health than you would otherwise. May you receive God's richest blessings and an understanding of the why of it. When the trials come, choose to prosper.

Other books written by Clive Buchanan

18 Steps to Greatness

Transfer Factor Against Inhuman Terrorists

Herbal Knowledge

Love, Money, and Personal Power

Walking With Lions

To order or get information about Books, CD's, cruises, products, or to hire Clive as a speaker call: 1-435-275-6649 or 1-888-344-3892 or e-mail: info@cjbuchanan.com

Chart & Journal to Better Health

Week beginning: _____

All Days	Mon	Tu	Wed	Thu	Fri	Sat	Sun	Success Days
Bee Pollen								
Transfer Factor								
Lecithin								
Gotu Kola								
L-Carnitine								
Siberian Ginseng								
Evening Primrose Oil								
Multiple Vitamins								
45 minute Exercise								
Played Mind Games								

Positive Outstanding Event of the Week:

_____

_____

_____

_____

Chart & Journal to Better Health

Week beginning: _____

All Days	Mon	Tu	Wed	Thu	Fri	Sat	Sun	Success Days
Bee Pollen								
Transfer Factor								
Lecithin								
Gotu Kola								
L-Carnitine								
Siberian Ginseng								
Evening Primrose Oil								
Multiple Vitamins								
45 Minute Exercise								
Played Mind Games								

Positive Outstanding Event of the Week:

_____

_____

_____

_____

_____

Chart & Journal to Better Health

Week beginning: _____

All Days	Mon	Tu	Wed	Thu	Fri	Sat	Sun	Success Days
Bee Pollen								
Transfer Factor								
Lecithin								
Gotu Kola								
L-Carnitine								
Siberian Ginseng								
Evening Primrose Oil								
Multiple Vitamins								
45 Minute Exercise								
Played Mind Games								

Positive Outstanding Event of the Week:

_____

_____

_____

_____

Chart & Journal to Better Health

Week beginning: _____

All Days	Mon	Tu	Wed	Thu	Fri	Sat	Sun	Success Days
Bee Pollen								
Transfer Factor								
Lecithin								
Gotu Kola								
L-Carnitine								
Siberian Ginseng								
Evening Primrose Oil								
Multiple Vitamins								
45 Minute Exercise								
Played Mind Games								

Positive Outstanding Event of the Week:

_____

_____

_____

_____

Chart & Journal to Better Health

Week beginning: _____

All Days	Mon	Tu	Wed	Thu	Fri	Sat	Sun	Success Days
Bee Pollen								
Transfer Factor								
Lecithin								
Gotu Kola								
L-Carnitine								
Siberian Ginseng								
Evening Primrose Oil								
Multiple Vitamins								
45 Minute Exercise								
Played Mind Games								

Positive Outstanding Event of the Week:

_____

_____

_____

_____

Chart & Journal to Better Health

Week beginning: _____

All Days	Mon	Tu	Wed	Thu	Fri	Sat	Sun	Success Days
Bee Pollen								
Transfer Factor								
Lecithin								
Gotu Kola								
L-Carnitine								
Siberian Ginseng								
Evening Primrose Oil								
Multiple Vitamins								
45 Minute Exercise								
Played Mind Games								

Positive Outstanding Event of the Week:

_____

_____

_____

_____